Herbal Remedies for Weight Loss

Burn Fat and Boost Your Metabolism with Herbs

I0427661

Disclaimer

Summary

'You need to lose weight,', say that statement to someone and you will get the same reaction every time. Weight loss is indeed a very serious problem growing rapidly with time. People around the world are doing different things to control their weight including dieting, exercising and taking medication.

Unfortunately, medication isn't a natural way and thus brings with it many side effects. However, alternative medicine is always available to become your weight loss solution. Yes, we are talking about herbs and herbal remedies for effective weight loss.

While diet and physical activity play an active role in reducing weight and weight management, doing it together by following some effective weight loss herbal remedies can give you better and long-lasting results.

What this book will provide you:

1. The reasons why extra weight can be a risk to your life
2. The non-herbal, quick home-remedies to help you get started with a healthy lifestyle
3. An introduction to a list of effective herbs for weight loss
4. Usage of herbs to deal with different weight-related health problems such as diabetes and poor digestion
5. Herbal recipes to deal with weight-related health problems and body detoxification
6. Insights on magical kitchen herbs for healthy cooking
7. A variety of weight loss herbal recipes to achieve weight loss successfully

In short, this book has all the information you need about herbs and herbal remedies for weight loss to help you get started. Read on and make a difference to your health and life!

Contents

Introduction: Battling the Bulge

Alternative Medicine – How Herbs Can Be Your Weight Loss Solution

Herbal solutions for weight loss are one of the most popular forms of alternative medication They are also the most commonly used, misused and, unfortunately, misunderstood.

These days, every other product claims to be the "natural" solution for weight loss. We are bombarded with a wide variety of products on TV, internet and even radio on a daily basis. A number of these products and supplements are presented cleverly, with herbal or natural weight loss ingredients' names and high prices.

In order to understand what herbs really are and how they can benefit us in achieving weight loss goals, you first need to avoid these false promises and gimmicks.. Instead, invest in organic, pure bulk herbs and follow home-made herbal remedies and formulas from them.

This way, you will not only be assured of the freshness and quality of the herbs you are consuming, but you will always have more than one way to fine-tune your weight loss formula and adjust it according to your own, individual metabolism.

Therefore, instead of relying on these packaged herbal supplements and weight loss teas, make your own without spending a fortune over the products that don't really work. Since you can rely on the quality of product you are using, you will get the full benefits of fat burning properties most of the herbs have. We will discuss about these herbs in detail later in this book.

Other Non-Herbal Home Remedies to Help Yourself Get Started

Before we jump to the herbal remedies for weight loss, follow these tips and tricks (non-herbal) to get yourself in the form. These home remedies will help you get started on this natural weight loss journey effectively.

You may believe that kitchen is the worst room in the house, especially when you are following a weight loss routine. This is not true. Staying out of the kitchen is not a cure if you are overweight. In fact, the kitchen is the place where you can begin losing weight. Work on creating a healthy kitchen before you begin.

Re-stocking your kitchen is one of the best home remedies to get yourself fat-reducing utensils and healthy food items that will help you lose weight.

It's time to stock up your kitchen with the best of herbs mentioned in this book and prepare amazing teas, smoothies and shakes using the weight loss herbal ingredients listed here. You will find some amazing recipes in this book that you can prepare at home. So keep reading and learn more about herbal remedies for weight loss.

Saying Goodbye to Fat Forever – Introducing the List of Effective Weight Loss Herbs

Weight problem? No problem! You are not the only one in this weight loss battle. For some it's cravings and a sedentary lifestyle, for others it could be a sluggish metabolism. Regardless of what your reason is, herbal formulas can work wonders for you.

Here is a list of the best herbs for weight loss. Keep reading, they could be your ultimate solution to achieving your weight loss goal:

Green Tea Extract

Green tea is made up of compounds known as catechins. These compounds belong to a class of antioxidants that are known for enhancing metabolism and boosting the ability to stimulate fat burning.

It was revealed in a study published in 2005 in the American Journal of Clinical Nutrition that a group of people were asked to consume 690 ml of green tea extract in a day along with diet control, while the other group only followed a controlled diet. At the end of three months, the first group that consumed green tea extract lost more weight in total. Studies also suggest that green tea extract is great for reducing weight, especially for women.

Green tea extract is a natural herb that is popular for its weight loss properties. It is also known for alleviating water retention in most cases.

Fish Oil

Fish oil contains Omega-3 fatty acids that are known for changing the body's behavior towards fat. Instead of using the fat to store it, the body burns it to generate energy. According to the American Journal of Clinical Nutrition, 2007, both exercise and fish oil independently can reduce body fat. But the combination of these two gave amazing results. Australian researchers suggested brisk walking for 45 minutes three times a week along with consuming 1.9 grams of fish oil on a daily basis.

It was also revealed that fish oil can significantly control your craving towards food, keeping you from unhealthy foods and gaining weight from unhealthy calories.

As far as consumption is concerned, it is suggested by experts to go slow with the dosage at first in order to avoid disrupting your sleep routine.

L-Glutamine

When your blood sugar level goes down, you start craving food because your brain requires more fuel. L-Glutamine, which is an amino acid, provides instant fuel to the brain, which immediately holds your cravings for starchy and sweet foods. Studies also show that L-Glutamine can facilitate weight loss by influencing the storage and conversion of calories.

According to a study held at Duke University Medical Center, supplements that included L-Glutamine caused mice to lose weight. L-Glutamine is now available in capsules too.

Gymnema Sylvestre

This herb comes from a plant native to the wild Africa and India. This herb has qualities to reduce the ability to taste sweetness. The molecules of gymnema are somewhat similar to glucose and can fill the taste bud receptors. The consumption of this herb will make you feel like you have gotten a sugar fix on your tongue.

In 1983, a study named Physiology and Behavior confirmed that people who regularly took gymnema had a weak perception of the sweet taste and, therefore, avoided sweet and snack foods and consumed fewer calories that helped them control their weight.

It is highly recommended to take gymnema in prescribed amounts to avoid low-blood sugar.

Guggul

Guggul is an Ayurvedic remedy known for boosting your metabolism and burning fat. The herb is also popular for lowering cholesterol, relieving joint pain and supporting weight loss. A research on guggul was held at the University of Nebraska in Omaha and at the Beth Israel Medical Center in New York City. A group of people were asked to take 750mg of guggul on a daily basis together with a combination of aerobic and strength training workout thrice a week and another group was only asked to follow the exercise routine. This routine was continually followed for six weeks.

At the end of the sixth week, the average weight loss for people who consumed guggul was 6 lbs whereas people who only followed the exercise routine lost ½ to 1 lb. The research concluded that guggul not only helps the body with metabolism, but also improves the function of the thyroid by enhancing the levels of thyroid hormones in the body.

Reishi Mushrooms

Reishi mushrooms grow on fallen logs and are usually harvested in the wild. These are commonly used as a major component of Traditional Chinese Medicine for immunity and strength to fight fatigue Reishi mushrooms are associated with weight loss because, according to nutritionists, to follow an exercise plan and a healthy diet routine, it is very important to feel energetic and strong.

Reishi mushrooms are also used to treat hypertension – one of the health hazards of being overweight or obese – through Traditional Chinese Medicine.

In addition to the above listed herbs, there is another long list of some popular herbs you might not have known could do wonders for your weight loss goal. Check them out below:

Cacao

Surprised at cacao? Well, according to studies, adults who consumed chocolate regularly are actually slimmer than people who avoid it completely and that regular, modest consumption of chocolate can be calorie-neutral.

Fennel Seed

Fennel seed is another famous name associated with weight loss. This ancient herb possesses the reputation as a weight loss solution and still holds it to date. Prepare yourself a cup of fennel seed tea and drink it 15-20 minutes before your meal. Wonderful results!

Chickweed

Chickweed or chickweed tea is also a popular and old remedy used by overweight and obese people to aid in weight loss. The herb also has blood cleansing-qualities and is a favorite among women, drank as a classic spring tonic to maintain health as well as weight.

Garcinia Fruit

Both extracted acid HCA and Garcinia Combogia are widely used to prepare weight loss herbal supplements. HCA slows down the formation of fatty acids resulting in less fat in the body for storage purposes. Studies have also revealed that HCA has appetite-controlling qualities. This herb can be used as prepared weight loss supplements in the form of tablets, powders, capsules and even snack bars. You can even follow the recipe to prepare a tea at home to aid in weight loss.

Grapefruit

Grapefruit can increase circulation, stimulating the lymphatic system and can also cleanse kidneys. Overall, grapefruit is an amazing solution to regular overall body weight if used on a regular basis.

Bladderwrack/Kelp

This is a very common herb, used in herbal medicines for thyroid stimulation and plays an effective role in weight loss if used as a part of diet regularly. Since it's a seaweed, there are other benefits associated with its consumption in addition to weight loss, such as cancer treatment.

Pomegranate

Pomegranates are loaded with punicic acid, which are a powerful form of CLA, known to be beneficial to fight against obesity, cancer, heart diseases and diabetes. Other than the high cost, there aren't any downsides associated with pomegranate. Add pomegranate or pomegranate juice to your daily diet.

Psyllium

The natural form of this herb can be your ultimate weight loss aid. Psyllium is your effective and safe weight loss herb that you can consume to boost your metabolism and burn fat. When consumed, the seed expands in your stomach, making you feel full and slowing down the process of simple carbohydrates absorption.

Green Tea

There are various studies proving the role of green tea in weight loss. Studies indicate that the consumption of green tea on a regular basis has amazing effects on your metabolic syndrome as well as weight loss.

Stevia

Stevia, used as an alternative to sugar, can have a significant impact on weight loss. Since the sweet leaves are used as a natural sweetener, it eliminates the requirement of sugar completely, ensuring less calorie consumption that helps in weight loss.

Yerba Mate

Yerba mate can be used as smooth caffeine. In addition, it is believed to have qualities to aid in weight loss by controlling food cravings and by helping you feel fuller for longer periods. The herb can be used to make various herbal weight loss recipes, which you can prepare at home for regular consumption.

Magical Kitchen Herbs for Healthy Cooking

There are so many beneficial things in your kitchen that you are probably unaware of. Your kitchen is loaded with powerful natural health remedies that you can use for your health. Culinary herbs such as thyme, sage and rosemary not only give flavor to foods when used while cooking, but also make your food healthy and full of benefits for your body.

Adding some common herbs like these to your diet supply vitamins, micronutrients and digestive enzymes to your food and add flavors to give your meal a great taste. Herbs can be thought of as both medicine and food.

The purpose of this book is to highlight all the herbal remedies that can be used with the medicinal aspect, especially for the purpose of weight loss. Other than herbs, there are food types and spices that have really blurred the distinction between medicine and food so much that they are considered almost the same thing. Some of these beneficial food items include honey, vinegar, onions, pepper and various spices.

Get your organic herbs from a nearby store or grow your own herbs at home right next to your kitchen window and make the most out of the health and weight loss benefits of these herbs. These herbs can be so eye-catching that just by looking at them you will feel inspired to eat and cook more healthy meals at home.

Recipes

Here are some amazing herbal recipes that you can make with ingredients present in your kitchen. Try these at home for weight loss and various other health benefits.

Cinnamon and Apple Vinegar

Use cinnamon to spice up apple vinegar and to prepare herbal blend that's not only healthy but delicious.

Ingredients

1 small Apple

Cinnamon, a small piece

Apple cider vinegar, 1-quart

Honey, ½ cups

Note: You can also use other fruits instead of apple such as cranberries, blackberries and raspberries.

Preparation Method

1. Cut one small apple into small chunks and place it in a clean container along with a small piece of cinnamon.
2. Set 1-quart apple cider vinegar over gentle heat. Add ½ cup honey and combine with the vinegar.
3. Add this vinegar to the container with apple chunks and cinnamon.
4. Stir and infuse for 1-2 weeks. Discard apple chunks, reserving the vinegar mixture with cinnamon.

Use this herbal vinegar for cooking healthy, delicious meals.

Cilantro Pesto

With a combination of garlic, nuts, cilantro and lemon juice, prepare organic and healthy cilantro pesto for amazing weight loss results.

Ingredients

Garlic (peeled), 1 clove

Almonds, brazil nuts or cashews (or a mix of these), ½ cup (finely chopped)

Fresh cilantro leaves (organic), 1 cup

Lemon juice (organic), 2 tbsp

Flax seed oil, 6 tbsp

Sea salt, to taste

Preparation Method

1. Pour flax seed oil and cilantro in a blender and pulse until the leaves are completely chopped.
2. Add nuts, garlic and lemon juice in the blender and blend again until the ingredients form a paste.
3. Add some salt and blend again to add flavors.
4. Store in a glass jar (dark) to use it for extended shelf life.

Basil Lemonade

Prepare a refreshing and uplifting summer drink with fresh and organic basil amply produced during the hot season. Complement the unique flavor of basil with mint or your own healthy variation for great results.

Ingredients

Fresh basil leaves (organic), ½ cup

Honey, 3 tbsp

Water, 4 cups

Lemon or limejuice, ½ cup

Preparation Method

1. Muddle honey and basil together.
2. Add water
3. Blend in citrus juice
4. Combine all ingredients thoroughly and allow infusion for at least 20 minutes.
5. Strain and add ice.
6. Serve chilled.

Basil Summer Tea

Use the most common kitchen herb to prepare a herbal tea for great health benefits and weight loss. Use the fresh basil leaves to prepare a mildly stimulating and refreshing basil tea. Serve with ice or hot, as you like.

Ingredients:

Fresh basil (organic), a handful (chopped)
Lemon juice, 1 tsp
Stevia, a few drops

Note: Use variations to give your summer basil tea a unique flavor. Your options include lemon, cinnamon, thai, dark chocolate, etc.

Preparation Method

1. Place a handful of chopped fresh basil leaves in a hot cup of water.
2. Allow the leaves to infuse for a few minutes, until the tea is drinkable.
3. Add a few drops of stevia and stir.
4. Give your tea a final lemon (or your favorite variation) twist and serve.

Note: You can enjoy a warm basil tea or serve over with ice for an ice-tea version,

Managing and Preventing Health Risks Associated with Fat – Herbs to Control Diabetes

Diabetes is the most common side effect of being overweight or obese. If you have piled up extra kilos on your body, . Fortunately, the ravages of this condition on our health are very well documented.

While type 2 diabetes can be a result of unhealthy lifestyle decisions and bad health due to being overweight, it can be turned around by making the right decisions. However, this could be a little challenging. Things like these are easier said than done. Bad lifestyle decisions and habits such as alcohol consumption or eating too much junk and fast food are extremely addictive and very difficult to overcome.

In such situations, herbs can be your amazing allies. Fighting diabetes is as important as fighting weight loss itself. Even if you are not suffering from diabetes currently, using herbs on a regular basis can benefit you in various aspects such as curbing sugar cravings and encouraging cooking at home to enjoy flavorful meals.

There are various diabetic friendly foods such as baked goods that are prepared using healthy spices like stevia and cinnamon, which reduces the requirement for sugar. According to a recent study, cinnamon cassia (cinnamomum aromaticum) can effectively improve the levels of blood sugar in diabetic patients and helps control sugar cravings, which eventually aid in weight loss.

Botanicals like fenugreek and bitter melon can also be used together with medicinal therapy to treat and manage diabetes. Bitter melon is known for improving glucose tolerance and body's ability to utilize blood sugar.

In addition to this, burdrock root also plays a significant role in controlling the level of blood sugar in the body since it's loaded with insulin content. In case you are already taking hypoglycemic drugs or insulin to maintain your blood sugar levels, make sure you speak with your doctor before starting any herbal treatment.

Recipes

Here are a few herbal recipes for both treating diabetes and effectively achieving weight loss goals. Read on.

Bitter Melon Tea

Prepare a healthy tea with dried bitter melon powder or slices. This tea has a nutty, mild flavors and a very pleasant taste. Add raw (organic) honey if you wish to sweeten it a bit.

Ingredients:

Dried bitter melon, 4 or 5 slices or 1 tsp powder

Preparation Method:

1. You may use slices of dried melon or melon powder (1 tsp), as you like.
2. Add to one cup of hot water.
3. Let is infuse for a few minutes until the tea is of drinkable temperature.

Note: Don't forget to consult your medical professional or healthcare provider for the right dosage of this tea if you are under cholesterol or diabetes treatment.

Burdock Herbal Tea

From treating diabetes to detoxification and skin benefits, burdock herbal tea can be your ultimate herbal solution for various problems. Make your own at home now.

Ingredients:

Burdock (dried root), 1 tbsp

Preparation Method:

1. Simmer the dried root in 2 cups of hot water.
2. Let it simmer for at least 20 minutes.
3. Drink up to four cups in a day.

Note: Ask your healthcare provider for the right dosage if you are under any medical treatment. The tea can also be used as a face and skin wash. When cooled, use a clean facecloth to apply the tea to the skin and rinse with clean, cool water

Honey and Cinnamon Blend

Cinnamon does not only add a unique flavor to any tea, it can be the perfect blend for any tea combination due to its warm, spicy properties. Use honey to add natural sweetness to the tea and drink for various health benefits.

Ingredients

Cinnamon chips (organic), 1 tsp for 1 cup of water
Raw honey, 1 tbsp

Preparation Method:

1. Add cinnamon to 1 cup of hot water.
2. Let it simmer for at least 10 minutes (covered).
3. Stir in 1 tbsp of honey.
4. Sprinkle ground cinnamon on top before drinking.

Carob Tea

An amazing tea with amazing results! A cup of carob tea after each meal can slow down the release of sugars into the blood stream. It also helps to curb the cravings for sugar and sugar-laden desserts.

Ingredients:

Carob pods (roasted and chopped), 1 tbsp
Raw honey, 1 tbsp

Note: To add flavor to this tea, do not hesitate in blending it with spices, orange and mint for a tasty, soothing tea.

Preparation Method:

1. Add carob pods in one cup of water.
2. Bring to a slow boil in a pan (covered).
3. Turn off stove and let it sit for 5 minutes
4. Drink hot for best results.

Dealing with Digestion Problems – Herbs to Cure Bloating, Gas and Poor Digestion

Poor digestion, bloating and gas are also some of the not-so-wanted gifts of being overweight and/or obese. If you are carrying extra body weight, it will surely affect your metabolism as well as your digestion process.

The good news is that there are various herbal home remedies which can help you with weight loss as well as treat your poor digestion and occasional heartburn. A poor digestive system is actually a chronic condition that requires a holistic and serious approach that treats the causes instead of the symptoms.

Relying on mainstream medicines mainly concentrates on controlling stomach acid for relieving symptoms of gas and heartburn but it also interferes with the digestion process, not letting the food we consume to be converted into usable energy for the body.

When discussing the herbs for digestion, mint teas and chamomile will surely top the list. Chamomile is known for relieving spasms, reducing inflammation and giving quick relief to bloating and gas. As far as mint herbs are concerned, the best choices to relieve vomiting, nausea sand support the gall bladder include bee balm, basil, spearmint and peppermint.

Lemon balm such as chamomile can have soothing results for treating nervous stomach disorders.

Aromatic Spices and Seeds

Herbs known for preventing bloating and dispelling gas are called carminatives. A majority of these are closely associated with the members of Apiaceae family. These aromatic spices and seeds help speed digestion and add enjoyment and flavor to our food.

These include the following:

1. Ajwain seed
2. Asafetida root
3. Anise seed
4. Black pepper
5. Cardamom
6. Caraway seed
7. Coriander
8. Dill
9. Cumin
10. Parsley
11. Fennel seed

The painful effects of bloating and poor digestion go far beyond just a stomachache. In fact, it is just the beginning of gastrointestinal conditions that, fortunately, can be treated with nutritional foods and herbs.

What you don't know is that a number of other root causes of bad health and excess weight begin with our food choices and how willing we are to convert that food into fuel for our body. Again, a poor metabolism is associated with a number of diseases including weight gain, chronic fatigue, rheumatoid arthritis and skin disorders.

Kitchen Cures

There are various natural digestive stimulants that you can use while cooking for boosted metabolism. Focus on your lifestyle and eating decisions and turn your food to produce fuel for your body instead of storing it as fat.

Add onions, garlic, leeks, shallots, chives and scallions for improved digestibility of heavy foods such as meats. Sage, savory and lemongrass are also known as culinary herbs that prevent indigestion and add flavor to the food. Cayenne and other types of peppers lessen the bloating and gas that results from greasy, heavy foods. Adding mustard to your food can boost the digestion process for fatty foods such as pork.

Recipes

These are some recipes to boost the digestion process and relieve gas and bloating. The benefits of these herbal remedies will eventually help you with weight loss.

Angelica Aromatic Bitter

The angelica roots are an excellent carminative and tonic. The infusion will immediately treat flatulence and stomach-aches. Use this aromatic bitter herb to also treat various digestive problems as well as weight loss.

Ingredients

Angelica root (chopped), 1 tsp
Orange peel (dried), 1 tsp
Fennel seeds, 1 tsp
Raw honey, 1 tbsp

Preparation Methods

1. In 2 cups of water, add one tablespoon of herb-mix.
2. Set over low-med heat and boil. Let the mixture simmer over low heat (covered) for 5-10 minutes.
3. Drink the mixture when warm, before or after meals.
4. Add a little raw honey for a sweet taste.

Bee Balm Tea

This American garden delight is the bees' favorite. A not very popular member of the mint family actually offers great benefits for digestion problems and weight loss issues.

Ingredients

Bee balm, a handful of leaves
Raw honey, 1 tbsp

Preparation Method

1. Infuse a handful of chopped fresh bee balm leaves in a hot cup of water.
2. Drink when the temperature of the tea is drinkable.

Bittersweet Blend for Stomach

Fennel and caraway are the dynamic duo that offers amazing benefits for stomach distress.

Ingredients

Caraway seed, 1 tsp
Fennel seed, 1 tsp
Dried yarrow flowers, 1 tsp
Dried wormwood leaf, 1 tsp

Preparation Method

1. Combine all the herbs in equal parts.
2. Crush the seeds to extract active principles.
3. Add one tsp of leaf and seed blend in boiling water.
4. Let it infuse for 15-20 minutes.
5. Drink when hot a few minutes before eating heavy meals.

Cardamom Tea

Cardamom tea is fragrant, warm and pleasant for taste buds. Use this light taste tea to prepare a tea to soothe your stomach problems.

Ingredients

Cardamom seeds, 1 tsp
Raw honey, 1 tsp
Cinnamon powder, a pinch

Preparation Method

1. Add cardamom seeds to hot water.
2. Let it infuse for a few minutes.
3. Stir in honey for sweetener.
4. Sprinkle a pinch of cinnamon powder.
5. Drink hot for best results.

Herbal Detoxification for Natural Weight Loss – Time for Herbal Cleanse

The best and most popular herbs for natural detoxification herbal cleanse includes chicory root, boldo, dandelion root, cypress oil, juniper berries, sassafras root and Oregon grape root. These herbal teas and baths are used for detoxification and are widely used for treating various chronic conditions that react to toxins within the body.

The herbs are beneficial for symptoms of acne breakouts, skin rashes, allergies, arthritis and others. Regular usage of these herbs will also benefit liver in purifying it. Poor health and weight gain also leads to poor liver function.

In order to achieve weight loss, it is important to treat these symptoms using herbal methods. Detoxifying or depurative herbs help cleanse toxins and waste from our body. These herbal options are a staple of conventional herbal medicines.

Recipes

If you are looking for natural herbal detoxification, here are some recipes to help you with that.

American Liver Tonic

The classics of native America such as dandelion, wild ginger and sassafras complement each other in action as well as taste. This tonic is beneficial for anyone who wishes to cleanse their system with natural herbs. Drink this soothing detoxifying blend early in the morning for great results.

Ingredients

Dandelion root (dried, chopped), 1 tsp
Sassafras root bark (dried, chopped), 1 tsp
Wild ginger root (dried, chopped), 1 tsp
1 clove
Honey, ½ tbsp

Preparation Method

1. Add dandelion root, sassafras root bark and wild ginger root powder to one cup of water and boil over low heat.
2. Remove from the stove and let it stand for 18-20 minutes (covered).
3. Before drinking, add 1 clove and ½ tbsp of honey and drink warm.

Note: This herbal tonic is not for consecutive use on a long term basis.

Blood Purification Tea

Purify and detoxify the blood with this interesting strong blend of wormwood and peppermint. In case the wormwood cannot be swallowed due to its strong bitter taste, reduce it.

Ingredients

Burdock, 2 parts
Nettle, 1 part
Peppermint, 1 part
Wormwood, ½ part (reduce further if you like)

Preparation Method

1. Add all the ingredients in one cup water and bring to boil over low med heat.
2. Pour it in a cup and let it cool a bit.
3. Add a hint of stevia or honey if the tea is too bitter to adjust taste.

Drink once a day for excellent results.

Rosemary and Ginger Bath

The combination of ginger and rosemary makes a soothing bath for arthritis pain, fibromyalgia and sore muscles. This bath is also detoxifying and depurative.

Ingredients

Rosemary essential oil, 6 drops
Fresh ginger (grated), 1 tbsp
Fresh rosemary sprigs, a few

Preparation Method

1. Prepare ginger tea by adding 1 tablespoon of fresh grated ginger to 1 ½ cups of warm water.
2. Stir, strain and add the ginger tea to bath water.
3. Add rosemary essential oil to the bath water as well.
4. Lastly, add fresh rosemary sprigs into the bath water and take a refreshing, soothing bath.

Red Clover Tea

Read clover tea comes with various health benefits for you. This herbal drink not only helps you with liver purification, it calms menstruation and menopause-related problems as well as treats skin problems naturally. It is an amazing herbal drink for women. While the taste isn't very pleasant, you can always blend it with other minty or citrusy herbs to enjoy better flavor.

Ingredients

Red Clover (dried leaves and flowers), 1 tsp
Peppermint, optional

Preparation Method

1. Add 1 tsp of dried herb to prepare1 cup of hot water.
2. Infuse for 5 minutes and drink.
3. Add peppermint if you wish to add a minty taste to your tea.

Herbal Recipes for Weight Loss

Here comes the part you have been waiting for – the most desirable, easy-to-prepare and result-yielding recipes for weight loss. Most of the recipes compiled here can be prepared with ingredients present at home. Move one step forward to achieve your weight loss goal with the help of these amazing herbal recipes for weight loss.

Chickweed Tea

Chickweed tea is a traditional yet effective remedy for weight loss. Chickweed does not only offer weight loss benefits and add a healthy ingredient to your diet plan, it also possesses the ability to purify blood and calm inflammation. Try making this at home and aid weight loss.

Ingredients

Chickweed, 1-2 tsp

Preparation Method

1. Add 1-2 tsp dried chickweed herb into 1 cup water.
2. Stir and bring it to boil.
3. Pour in a cup and allow cooling for 5 minutes.
4. Drink warm or cool, as you like.

Note: Cooled chickweed tea is known to have anti-inflammatory effects to cure skin irritations and rashes.

Acai Berry Smoothie

Prepare an amazing antioxidant smoothie that offers great weight loss benefits. Use acai freeze dried powder as your main ingredient. This delicious drink can be enjoyed as an afternoon pick or along with the breakfast in the morning.

Ingredients

Acai powder, 1 tbsp

1 medium-sized ripe banana

Yogurt, 1 cup

Almond flavor, 1 tsp

Soymilk, 1 cup

Ice, ½ cup

Preparation Method

1. Add all ingredients to an electric blender one by one.
2. Pulse to blend until smooth.
3. Add ice in the end for great results.
4. Serve chilled.

Note: if you wish to avoid ice, use frozen banana or yogurt for your smoothie.

Fennel Seed Tea

Prepare a pleasant tasting, licorice-flavored tea with fennel seeds. While the tea has a great flavor by itself, you can always blend with other herbs for a flavorful addition. Known as an effective weight loss tea, fennel seed tea also helps with poor digestion, bloating and gas problems. One cup of this tea after a heavy meal could be your most effective and simplest remedy for weight loss.

Ingredients

Fennel seeds, 1 tsp
Ajawin seeds, ½ tsp (optional)

Preparation Method

1. Bruise the fennel seeds using a mortar.
2. Pestle the seeds to extract essential oil right before you set it to brew.
3. Infuse 1 teaspoon in each cup of boiling water for 10 minutes with lid on the vessel.
4. Strain well and serve hot.

Note: A cup of fennel seed tea when consumed half an hour before meals can help reduce your appetite and hence can result in effective weight loss.

Mate and Damiana Tea for Weight Loss

A weight loss blend made by mate and damiana works to help burn fat by boosting your metabolism. Add lemongrass to the blend for added flavor.

Ingredients

Damiana, 1 part

Mate, 1 part

White willow bark, ½ part

lemongrass, optional

Cinnamon, optional

Preparation method

1. Add the herbs into hot water and let it sit for a few minutes.
2. Strain and add your favorite flavors (lemongrass or cinnamon).
3. Add ½ tsp honey or a few drops of Stevia for added flavor.
4. Serve hot and fresh.

Note: This blend can be consumed up to three times a day before meals to boost metabolism for faster fat burn. Drink according to the directions for amazing results!

Red and Green Tea Break

Green tea and rooibos – this blend of red and green tea combination is loaded with delicious antioxidant that will greatly help you with your weight loss. Prepare and relish during afternoon or as a great mid-day pick up. For a natural sweetener, use stevia instead of honey and burn calories.

Ingredients

Green tea, 1 tsp

Rooibos, 1 tsp

Stevia, a few drops

Cinnamon, optional

Preparation Method

1. Steep the herbs into hot water.
2. Strain within 2-3 minutes to avoid bitterness.
3. Add stevia and stir
4. For additional flavor, you may even add a dash of cinnamon.
5. Enjoy hot for amazing calorie burning results.

Garcinia and Hibiscus Fat Loss Recipe

Prepare this diet tea using two famous herbs easily available in extract form – garcinia fruit and bitter orange. At a grocery store, garcinia fruit is commonly known as "garcinia cambogia," so don't get confused.

Ingredients

Bitter orange (dried), 1 tbsp

Garcinia, 2 medium-sized pieces

Fennel seeds, 1 tsp

Raw honey, ½ tsp

Preparation Method

1. Add all the herbs into a 1 ½ quart of cold water.
2. Cook at low - med heat and bring to boil.
3. Allow to simmer for a few minutes at low heat.
4. Strain and add ½ tsp honey for a sweet flavor.
5. Serve hot

Note: This tea could be pucker your mouth sour as it is extremely astringent. Therefore, make sure you adjust the natural sweetener accordingly.

Hibiscus and Garcinia Fat Burner Tea

Prepare the amazing hibiscus and garcinia burgundy blend and serve yourself with the perfect weight loss tea. Both of these main ingredients are a great source of HCA, which is an acid present in various diet supplements. When consumed in tea form, the benefits could be much more than just weight loss.

Ingredients

Hibiscus, 1 tbsp

Dried garcinia fruit, 2 small-sized pieces

Fresh ginger (grated), 3 tbsp

Hawthorn berry, 1 tbsp

Lemon slice

A few drops of stevia

Preparation Method

1. In 4 cups of cold water, add all the herbs.
2. Cover with tight lid and cook in a non-reactive pan.
3. Bring the mixture to a boil over low heat.
4. Reduce heat and simmer for 15-20 minutes.
5. Strain and add lemon slice and stevia.
6. Stir and serve hot or with ice, as you like.

Note: Not suitable for children younger than 12 years.

Hibiscus Tea

Make a pleasant-looking tea using hibiscus, which is loaded in trace minerals, antioxidants and vitamin C. This tea is considered very healthy for your entire family because not only it helps people losing weight to achieve their goals; it also helps control blood pressure naturally.

Ingredients

Hibiscus (dried), 1 tsp
Lemon, a few drops
Raw honey, ½ tsp

Preparation Method

1. Add 1 tsp of dried hibiscus herb into one cup of hot water.
2. Infuse for 10 minutes in a covered container.
3. Add lemon and stir.
4. Add raw honey and stir.
5. Serve cold or hot, as you like.

Ginger and Hibiscus Tea

Ginger and hibiscus are two tastes that complement each other greatly. Add it as your favorite summer drink and aid your weight loss naturally with natural herbs.

Ingredients

Dried hibiscus, 1 tbsp

Fresh grated ginger, 1 tbsp

Water, 4 cups

Stevia, a few drops

Mint, ½ tsp

Preparation Method

1. Combine all herbs in a large container.
2. Pour boiling water on the top and let it sit for 12-15 minutes.
3. The color will change to a beautiful ruby red.
4. Add stevia and stir.
5. Serve cold over ice or hot and add a sprig of mint for delicious taste.

Honeybush Tea

Honeybush is a caffeine-free, healthy tea loaded with magnesium, calcium, potassium and vitamin c. Prepare this tea at home and add to your diet routine for amazing results.

Ingredients

Honeybush, 2 tsp

Fresh ginger (grated), ½ tsp

Raw honey, ½ tsp

Lemon, a few drops

Preparation Method

1. Infuse 2 tsp of honeybush in one cup of hot water.
2. Strain and add ginger, honey and lemon.
3. Stir and serve hot.
4. For summer, serve with iced tea and make it an amazing refreshing summer blend.

Blends of Yerba Mate for Fat Burning

If you wish to make a healthy, delicious and smooth tea, this one's for you. It tastes so mild and smooth that you can easily overindulge. However, keep calm and don't forget it's a weight loss drink!

Ingredients

Yerba mate, 1 part

Hibiscus, 1 part

Raw honey, ½ tsp

Lemon, a few drops

Preparation Method

1. Combine the herbs.
2. Pour hot (not boiling) water over the leave and herbs.
3. Infuse for at least 15-20 minutes in a covered container.
4. Add honey and lemon and stir for flavoring.
5. Garnish with fresh mint and serve hot.

Super Green Shake

This delicious and light smoothie is loaded with high quality protein to help you with your weight loss goal and provide you with required nutrition.

Ingredients

Almond milk, 8 oz

Banana (frozen), 1 medium-sized

Ice cubes, a few

Protein powder, 1 tbsp

Barley grass powder, 1 tbsp

Preparation Method

1. Slice a medium-sized banana and set it to freeze for a few hours.
2. Add almond milk, ice cubes, protein powder and frozen banana in an electric blender.
3. Pulse at high until smooth.
4. Drink and enjoy chilled!

Final Word

We have compiled some of the best and easiest-to-make recipes in this book for you. We hope you like and enjoy the herbal remedies for weight loss shared in this book and use the information provided to achieve your weight loss goal.

Most of the recipes are prepared with easily available herbs and ingredients, most of which are usually present at home. So this could be your simple and pocket-friendly way to get to your ideal weight this time.

Make the most out of the information available in this book and make your weight loss journey natural and enjoyable.

Good luck!